Dr Patrick Wisedoc

Epilepsy:
Understanding, Managing, and Living Well

Epilepsy: Understanding, Managing, and Living Well

"Knowing your illness early can save you much suffering."

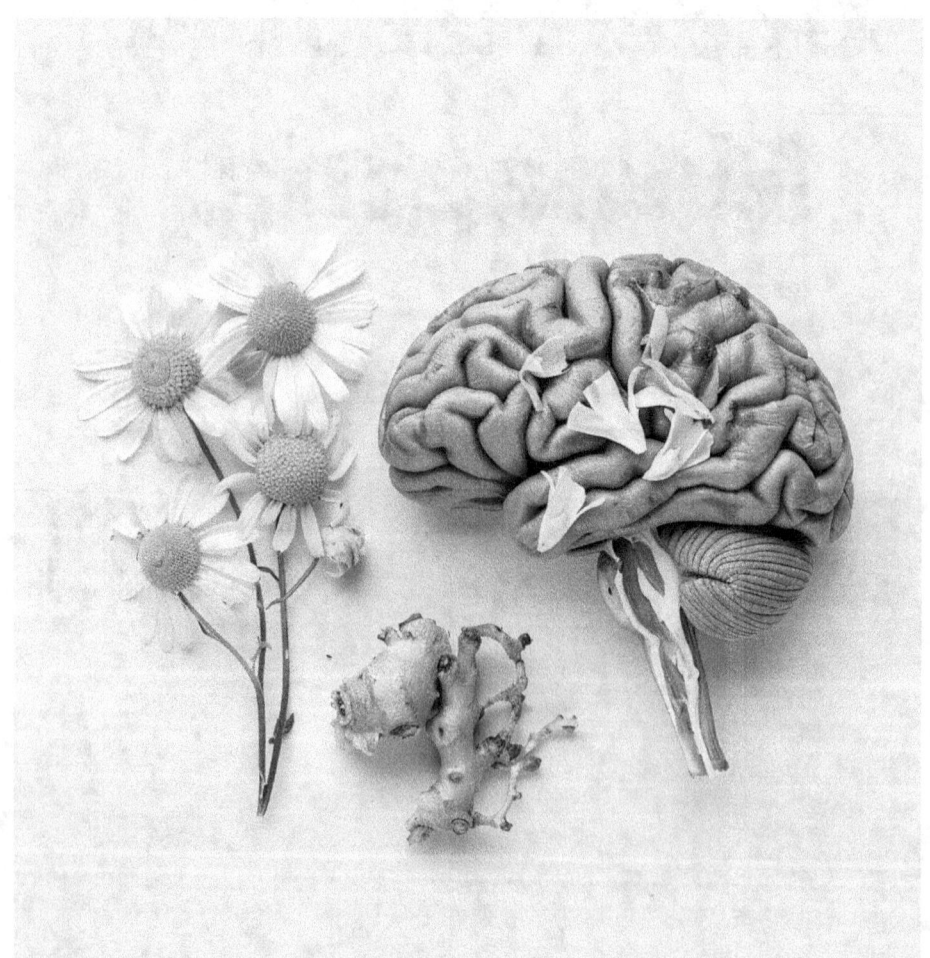

Introduction

Epilepsy: Understanding, Managing, and Living Well

Epilepsy can be a daunting topic, but understanding the condition and the options available can empower you to live a fulfilling life. This guide will explore epilepsy from various angles, providing valuable information on:

- **Understanding Seizures and Epilepsy:** We'll break down the causes, types, and effects of seizures, helping you gain a clear picture of the condition.
- **Managing Seizures:** Explore effective strategies for managing seizures, including medication, lifestyle changes, and self-management techniques.
- **Natural and Complementary Approaches:** While not a replacement for medical treatment, we'll explore complementary approaches like stress management and healthy habits that may support your overall well-being.
- **Living Well with Epilepsy:** Discover how to navigate the social and emotional aspects of epilepsy, building a strong support system and maintaining a positive outlook.
- **The Future of Epilepsy Treatment:** Exciting advancements in research offer hope for improved treatments and even potential cures.

This comprehensive guide aims to equip you with the knowledge and resources you need to manage epilepsy effectively and live a healthy, fulfilling life.

Contents

Part 1: Understanding Epilepsy

Chapter 1: What is Epilepsy?

- Subsection 1.1: Definition and Types of Seizures
- Subsection 1.2: Causes and Risk Factors
- Subsection 1.3: Diagnosis of Epilepsy

Chapter 2: Living with Epilepsy (combines "Epilepsy Syndromes" and "How Will Epilepsy Affect My Life?")

- Subsection 2.1: Types of Epilepsy Syndromes
- Subsection 2.2: Social, Emotional, and Cognitive Impact

Part 2: Managing Seizures

Chapter 3: Understanding Seizures

- Subsection 3.1: Different Types of Seizures (goes into more detail here)

Chapter 4: Responding to Seizures

- Subsection 4.1: Self-Management Strategies During a Seizure
- Subsection 4.2: Family Management Strategies During a Seizure

Contents

Chapter 5: Controlling Seizures

- Subsection 5.1: General Treatment Considerations
- Subsection 5.2: The Role of Nutrition in Epilepsy (dietary approaches and consulting a nutritionist)

Part 3: Natural and Complementary Approaches

Chapter 6: Natural Therapies for Epilepsy

- Subsection 6.1: Importance of Evidence-Based Practices

Chapter 7: Exploring Specific Natural Approaches

- Subsection 7.1: Herbal Remedies for Epilepsy (safety and research focus)
- Subsection 7.2: Vitamin Supplementation (refer to consulting a doctor)
- Subsection 7.3: Lifestyle Changes for Seizure Control (stress management, sleep hygiene, exercise)

Chapter 8: Alternative Therapies for Epilepsy

- Subsection 8.1: Acupuncture
- Subsection 8.2: Massage
- Subsection 8.3: Mind-Body Approaches (meditation, yoga)

Contents

Part 4: Living Well with Epilepsy

Chapter 9: Importance of Sleep (combines "Sleep and Epilepsy")

- Chapter 10: Understanding Seizure Effects
- Subsection 10.1: Breathing and Autonomic Disturbances
- Subsection 10.2: Consequences of Seizures (cognitive and other long-term effects)

Chapter 11: Self-Management for Epilepsy (combines "Self-Management Strategies in Epilepsy" and "Coping with Epilepsy")

- Subsection 11.1: Techniques for Managing Your Condition
- Subsection 11.2: Emotional and Social Support (including support groups and mental health considerations)

Part 5: The Future of Epilepsy Treatment

Chapter 12: Looking Ahead: Future Treatments and Technologies

Part 1: Understanding Epilepsy

Chapter 1: What is Epilepsy?

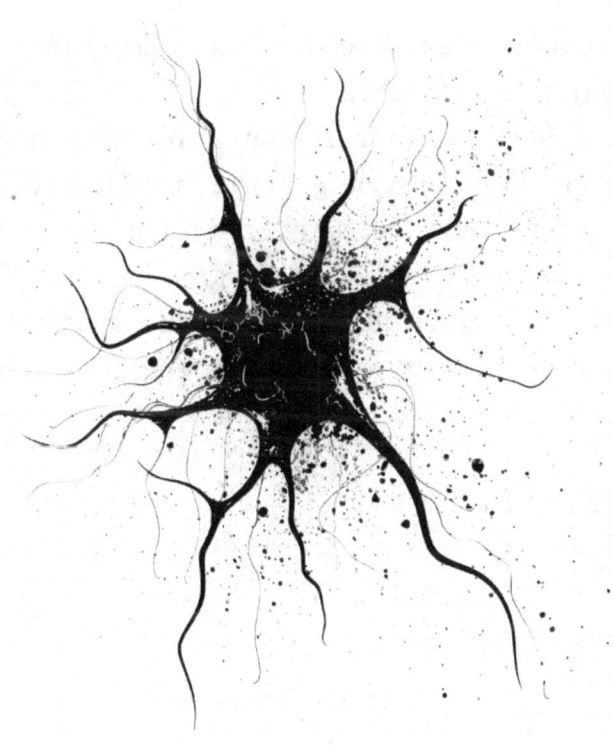

Part 1: Understanding Epilepsy
Chapter 1: What is Epilepsy?

Epilepsy is a chronic neurological disorder characterized by recurrent seizures. It's important to understand that a single seizure doesn't necessarily mean someone has epilepsy. Typically, two or more unprovoked seizures (meaning they occur without a clear trigger) are needed for an epilepsy diagnosis.

Here's a breakdown of key aspects of epilepsy:

- **Brain Activity:** Epilepsy results from abnormal electrical activity in the brain. This disrupts how brain cells communicate, leading to the various symptoms associated with seizures.
- **Types of Seizures:** Seizures can manifest in a wide variety of ways, depending on the location and extent of the abnormal electrical activity in the brain. We'll explore different seizure types in detail in the next section.
- **Causes:** While the exact cause of epilepsy is unknown in some cases, there are various factors that can contribute to its development. These include:
  - Head injury
  - Stroke
  - Brain tumors
  - Genetic predisposition
  - Infections
  - Developmental brain abnormalities
  - Diagnosis: Diagnosing epilepsy involves a multi-step process typically including a detailed medical history, neurological examination, and brain imaging tests (like EEG - Electroencephalogram)

Part 1: Understanding Epilepsy
Chapter 1: What is Epilepsy?

Living with Epilepsy:

Epilepsy can be a challenging condition, but with proper treatment and management, many people with epilepsy can live fulfilling lives. There are various treatment options available, including medications, dietary approaches, and in some cases, surgery.

Part 1: Understanding Epilepsy
Chapter 1: What is Epilepsy?
Subsection 1.1: Definition and Types of Seizures

What is a Seizure?

Imagine your brain as a complex electrical network. Normally, these electrical signals flow smoothly, allowing you to think, move, and feel the world around you. A seizure disrupts this delicate balance. It's a sudden, uncontrolled burst of electrical activity that throws the brain's normal function into temporary chaos. This can manifest in a variety of ways, depending on the location and intensity of the electrical discharge. Seizures can be brief or last for several minutes, and their severity can range from mild to dramatic.

Unveiling the Different Types of Seizures

Epilepsy can manifest in a variety of seizure types, broadly classified into two main categories based on where the abnormal electrical activity originates in the brain:

1. Focal Onset Seizures (Previously called Partial Seizures):

These seizures start in a specific region of the brain. The symptoms you experience will depend on the location of the seizure activity. Here's a breakdown of some focal onset seizures:

Part 1: Understanding Epilepsy
Chapter 1: What is Epilepsy?
Subsection 1.1: Definition and Types of Seizures

- **Simple Partial Seizures:** These seizures don't affect consciousness. You might experience unusual sensations, emotions, movements, or even see strange lights, all localized to a particular area of your body. For instance, you might feel a tingling sensation in your arm or experience a sudden taste in your mouth.

- **Complex Partial Seizures:** These seizures cause a temporary alteration or complete loss of consciousness. You might appear confused, have difficulty speaking, or experience automatisms (unconscious repetitive movements like lip smacking or fumbling).

Part 1: Understanding Epilepsy
Chapter 1: What is Epilepsy?
Subsection 1.1: Definition and Types of Seizures

2. Generalized Onset Seizures:

These seizures begin with abnormal electrical activity that affects both hemispheres of the brain simultaneously. This widespread disruption typically causes a loss of consciousness and may involve convulsions (jerking movements). Here are some common types of generalized onset seizures:

- **Tonic-Clonic Seizures (Previously called Grand Mal Seizures):** These are the most dramatic type, causing stiffening of the body (tonic phase) followed by jerking movements (clonic phase) and a period of unconsciousness.

- **Absence Seizures:** These brief seizures (lasting seconds) cause a temporary lapse in awareness. You might appear blank or stare vacantly during the seizure.

- **Atonic Seizures:** These seizures cause a sudden loss of muscle tone, often leading to collapsing or dropping objects.

- **Myoclonic Seizures:** These are brief, jerking movements of a muscle or group of muscles.

Part 1: Understanding Epilepsy
Chapter 1: What is Epilepsy?
Subsection 1.1: Definition and Types of Seizures

Important Considerations:

Some seizures may start as focal onset and then spread to become generalized onset (secondary generalized seizures). This is not an exhaustive list of all seizure types. There are rarer variations as well.
Understanding the specific type of seizure someone experiences is crucial for diagnosis and treatment planning. The next section will explore the diagnostic process for epilepsy.

Part 1: Understanding Epilepsy
Chapter 1: What is Epilepsy?
Subsection 1.2: Causes and Risk Factors

Epilepsy can be a perplexing condition. While the exact cause remains a mystery in some cases, researchers have identified various factors that can contribute to its development. This section delves into the potential triggers that might spark a seizure.

Potential Causes of Epilepsy

The root cause of epilepsy can vary depending on the individual. Here are some common culprits:

- Brain Abnormalities: Developmental abnormalities in the brain structure, present from birth (congenital), can increase the risk of seizures. These abnormalities can affect how brain cells communicate.
- Head Injuries: Severe head trauma can damage brain tissue and disrupt electrical activity, potentially leading to epilepsy.
- Stroke: Strokes that damage areas of the brain responsible for electrical control can increase the risk of seizures.
- Infections: Infections that inflame the brain, such as meningitis or encephalitis, can cause temporary or long-term epilepsy.
- Brain Tumors: Tumors growing in the brain can disrupt normal electrical activity and trigger seizures.
- Genetic Predisposition: Having a family history of epilepsy increases the risk, although it's not a guaranteed inheritance.

Part 1: Understanding Epilepsy
Chapter 1: What is Epilepsy?
Subsection 1.2: Causes and Risk Factors

Risk Factors Beyond the Cause

While understanding the specific cause is important, it's equally crucial to be aware of risk factors that might increase your susceptibility to seizures. Here are some to consider:

- Age: Epilepsy can develop at any age, but it's most commonly diagnosed in young children and adults over 65.
- Febrile Seizures: Children who experience febrile seizures (convulsions triggered by a high fever) have a slightly higher risk of developing epilepsy later in life.
- Certain Medical Conditions: Some neurological disorders like Alzheimer's disease and metabolic disorders can increase the risk of seizures.
- Substance Abuse: Alcohol and drug abuse can disrupt brain function and trigger seizures.
- Sleep Deprivation: Chronic lack of sleep can lower the seizure threshold, making them more likely to occur.
- It's important to note that having a risk factor doesn't necessarily mean you'll develop epilepsy. However, being aware of these factors can help you make informed lifestyle choices and discuss any concerns with your doctor.

Part 1: Understanding Epilepsy
Chapter 1: What is Epilepsy?
Subsection 1.3: Diagnosis of Epilepsy

Epilepsy can be a challenging condition to diagnose, especially since a single seizure doesn't necessarily mean you have it. This section explores the steps involved in diagnosing epilepsy and achieving a clear understanding of your specific situation.

The Diagnostic Journey

Diagnosing epilepsy involves a multi-pronged approach, gathering various pieces of information to build a comprehensive picture. Here's a breakdown of the key steps:

- Detailed Medical History: Your doctor will ask about your medical history, including any past head injuries, infections, or neurological conditions. They'll also inquire about your family history of epilepsy and any potential triggers you've noticed before your seizures.

- Neurological Examination: A neurological exam will assess your nervous system function, including reflexes, coordination, balance, and cognitive abilities. This helps identify any abnormal neurological signs that might be associated with epilepsy.

Part 1: Understanding Epilepsy
Chapter 1: What is Epilepsy?
Subsection 1.3: Diagnosis of Epilepsy

- Brain Imaging Tests: Imaging tests like CT scans or MRIs can help identify any structural abnormalities in the brain that could be contributing to your seizures.

- Electroencephalogram (EEG): This is the most crucial test for epilepsy diagnosis. An EEG measures the electrical activity of your brain using electrodes placed on your scalp. While a normal EEG doesn't rule out epilepsy, abnormal patterns during an EEG recording can strongly suggest seizure activity. In some cases, an EEG may be recorded while you sleep (sleep EEG) or during a video-EEG monitoring session where your seizures are captured on video alongside the brain activity recording. This additional information helps doctors pinpoint the specific location of the seizure activity in the brain.

Part 1: Understanding Epilepsy
Chapter 1: What is Epilepsy?
Subsection 1.3: Diagnosis of Epilepsy

Additional Tests:

Depending on your specific situation, your doctor might recommend additional tests, such as blood tests to rule out infections or metabolic imbalances that could be mimicking epilepsy.

Reaching a Diagnosis:

After reviewing all the information gathered from your medical history, neurological exam, imaging tests, and EEG, your doctor will be able to determine if you have epilepsy and the specific type of epilepsy you might have. This diagnosis allows for the development of a personalized treatment plan.

Part 1: Understanding Epilepsy
Chapter 2: Living with Epilepsy
Subsection 2.1: Types of Epilepsy Syndromes

While we've explored the different types of seizures, epilepsy itself can be further categorized based on the specific patterns of seizures a person experiences, the underlying cause (if known), and the age of onset. These categories are called epilepsy syndromes.

Understanding your specific epilepsy syndrome can be helpful for both diagnosis and treatment planning. Here's a breakdown of some common epilepsy syndromes:

Childhood Epilepsy Syndromes:

- Childhood Absence Epilepsy: This syndrome typically starts between 4 and 10 years old and is characterized by frequent absence seizures (brief lapses in awareness).

- Benign Rolandic Epilepsy (BRE): This syndrome, also known as benign childhood epilepsy with centrotemporal spikes, usually begins between 5 and 10 years old. It mainly causes simple partial seizures affecting the face and mouth.

- West Syndrome: This syndrome affects infants and young children, causing a specific type of seizure called infantile spasms. These are short, intense seizures that often involve a sudden flexion of the body and limbs.

Part 1: Understanding Epilepsy
Chapter 2: Living with Epilepsy
Subsection 2.1: Types of Epilepsy Syndromes

Epilepsy Syndromes that Begin in Adolescence or Adulthood:

- **Juvenile Myoclonic Epilepsy:** This syndrome typically starts in adolescence and is characterized by myoclonic seizures (brief jerking movements) and sometimes generalized tonic-clonic seizures.

- **Mesial Temporal Lobe Epilepsy:** This syndrome arises from abnormal electrical activity in the temporal lobes of the brain. It can cause various seizure types, including simple partial seizures with auras (unusual sensations before a seizure), complex partial seizures, and sometimes generalized tonic-clonic seizures.

- **Febrile Seizure Plus (FS+):** This syndrome includes a history of febrile seizures (convulsions triggered by a fever) in childhood, followed by the development of other seizure types later in life.

Part 1: Understanding Epilepsy
Chapter 2: Living with Epilepsy
Subsection 2.1: Types of Epilepsy Syndromes

Other Epilepsy Syndromes:

There are many other epilepsy syndromes, each with its own unique characteristics and seizure types. Some syndromes may be related to specific genetic mutations or brain malformations.

Importance of Epilepsy Syndrome Classification:

Identifying your specific epilepsy syndrome helps your doctor:

- Tailor treatment: Different epilepsy syndromes may respond better to specific medications or other treatment approaches.

- Predict seizure types: Understanding the typical seizure types associated with your syndrome can help you and your loved ones be prepared.

- Provide a prognosis: Some epilepsy syndromes are more likely to improve with treatment than others.

Part 1: Understanding Epilepsy
Chapter 2: Living with Epilepsy
Subsection 2.2: Social, Emotional, and Cognitive Impact

Epilepsy can have a significant impact not just on the physical experience of seizures, but also on your social, emotional, and cognitive well-being. This section will explore these potential effects and offer strategies for navigating them.

Social Impact:

- Isolation and Stigma: The fear of having a seizure in public can lead to social withdrawal and isolation. Additionally, there may be a stigma associated with epilepsy, making it difficult to talk openly about the condition.

- Relationships and Activities: Epilepsy can affect your relationships with family, friends, and romantic partners. It might also limit your ability to participate in certain activities.

Emotional Impact:

- Anxiety and Fear: Living with the constant possibility of having a seizure can cause significant anxiety and fear.
- Depression and Frustration: The challenges of managing epilepsy can lead to feelings of depression and frustration.
- Low Self-Esteem: Epilepsy can negatively affect your self-esteem if you feel limited or defined by your condition.

Part 1: Understanding Epilepsy
Chapter 2: Living with Epilepsy
Subsection 2.2: Social, Emotional, and Cognitive Impact

Cognitive Impact:

- Memory and Learning Difficulties: Some types of epilepsy and certain medications can affect memory, concentration, and learning abilities.

- Slower Processing Speed: People with epilepsy may experience slower processing speed, impacting their ability to complete tasks quickly.

Strategies for Managing the Impact:

- Education and Open Communication: Educating yourself and others about epilepsy can help dispel myths and promote understanding. Open communication with loved ones about your condition and its impact can foster support.

- Support Groups: Connecting with others who understand the challenges of epilepsy can be invaluable. Support groups offer a safe space to share experiences and receive encouragement.

- Therapy: Talking to a therapist can help you develop coping mechanisms for anxiety, depression, and other emotional challenges related to epilepsy.

Part 1: Understanding Epilepsy
Chapter 2: Living with Epilepsy
Subsection 2.2: Social, Emotional, and Cognitive Impact

- Healthy Lifestyle: Maintaining a healthy lifestyle with regular sleep, exercise, and a balanced diet can improve your overall well-being and potentially help manage your seizures.

- Finding Your Voice: Advocating for yourself and raising awareness about epilepsy can empower you and contribute to a more inclusive environment.

Remember: You are not alone. There are resources available to help you manage the social, emotional, and cognitive impact of epilepsy. By being proactive and seeking support, you can live a fulfilling life despite the challenges of this condition.

Part 2: Managing Seizures

Chapter 3: Understanding Seizures

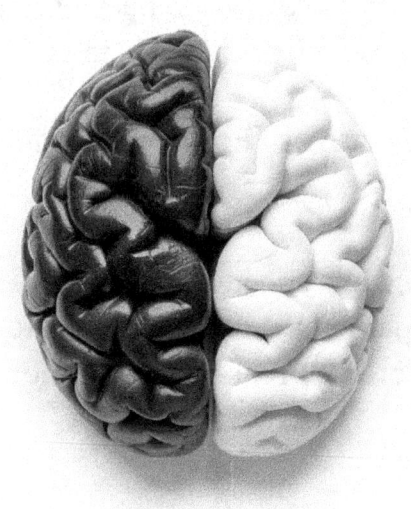

Part 2: Managing Seizures
Chapter 3: Understanding Seizures
Subsection 3.1: Different Types of Seizures

What is a Seizure?

Imagine your brain as a complex electrical network. Normally, these electrical signals flow smoothly, allowing you to think, move, and feel the world around you. A seizure disrupts this delicate balance. It's a sudden, uncontrolled burst of electrical activity that throws the brain's normal function into temporary chaos. This can manifest in a variety of ways, depending on the location and intensity of the electrical discharge. Seizures can be brief or last for several minutes, and their severity can range from mild to dramatic.

Unveiling the Different Types of Seizures
Epilepsy can manifest in a variety of seizure types, broadly classified into two main categories based on where the abnormal electrical activity originates in the brain:

1. Focal Onset Seizures (Previously called Partial Seizures):

These seizures start in a specific region of the brain. The symptoms you experience will depend on the location of the seizure activity. Here's a breakdown of some focal onset seizures:

Part 2: Managing Seizures
Chapter 3: Understanding Seizures
Subsection 3.1: Different Types of Seizures

- **Simple Partial Seizures:** These seizures don't affect consciousness. You might experience unusual sensations, emotions, movements, or even see strange lights, all localized to a particular area of your body. For instance, you might feel a tingling sensation in your arm or experience a sudden taste in your mouth.

- **Complex Partial Seizures:** These seizures cause a temporary alteration or complete loss of consciousness. You might appear confused, have difficulty speaking, or experience automatisms (unconscious repetitive movements like lip smacking or fumbling).

Part 2: Managing Seizures
Chapter 3: Understanding Seizures
Subsection 3.1: Different Types of Seizures

2. Generalized Onset Seizures:

These seizures begin with abnormal electrical activity that affects both hemispheres of the brain simultaneously. This widespread disruption typically causes a loss of consciousness and may involve convulsions (jerking movements). Here are some common types of generalized onset seizures:

- **Tonic-Clonic Seizures (Previously called Grand Mal Seizures):** These are the most dramatic type, causing stiffening of the body (tonic phase) followed by jerking movements (clonic phase) and a period of unconsciousness.

- **Absence Seizures:** These brief seizures (lasting seconds) cause a temporary lapse in awareness. You might appear blank or stare vacantly during the seizure.

- **Atonic Seizures:** These seizures cause a sudden loss of muscle tone, often leading to collapsing or dropping objects.

- **Myoclonic Seizures:** These are brief, jerking movements of a muscle or group of muscles.

Part 2: Managing Seizures
Chapter 3: Understanding Seizures
Subsection 3.1: Different Types of Seizures

Important Considerations:

- Some seizures may start as focal onset and then spread to become generalized onset (secondary generalized seizures).
- This is not an exhaustive list of all seizure types. There are rarer variations as well.
- Understanding the specific type of seizure someone experiences is crucial for diagnosis and treatment planning. The next section will explore the diagnostic process for epilepsy.

Part 2: Managing Seizures
Chapter 4: Responding to Seizures
4.1: Self-Management Strategies During a Seizure

A seizure can be a frightening experience, both for the person having it and for those witnessing it. However, by being prepared and knowing what to do, you can minimize risks and ensure the person's safety during a seizure. This section focuses on self-management strategies for individuals with epilepsy, along with crucial tips for bystanders.

For People with Epilepsy:

- Be Aware of Your Triggers: Identifying and avoiding seizure triggers, such as sleep deprivation, stress, or certain medications, can significantly reduce your risk of experiencing a seizure.

- Wear a Medical Alert Bracelet: A medical alert bracelet can provide vital information to first responders in case of a seizure occurring in public.

- Have a Seizure Action Plan: Develop a personalized seizure action plan with your doctor. This plan should outline what to do before, during, and after a seizure, and should be shared with loved ones, teachers, or colleagues.

- Carry Emergency Medication: If prescribed by your doctor, carry emergency medication (e.g., rescue medications) readily available to use during a seizure, if appropriate. It's crucial to follow your doctor's specific instructions regarding medication use.

Part 2: Managing Seizures
Chapter 4: Responding to Seizures
4.1: Self-Management Strategies During a Seizure

During a Seizure:

- Stay Calm: If you feel an aura (warning sensation) before a seizure, try to find a safe place to sit or lie down.
- Protect Yourself: If possible, move away from any hazards like sharp objects or hot surfaces to prevent injuries during the seizure.
- Focus on Breathing: Try to relax and focus on slow, deep breaths if you're conscious.

Important Note:

It's not recommended to try to restrain someone during a seizure. This can actually cause injuries.

For Bystanders Witnessing a Seizure:

- Stay Calm: The most important thing is to remain calm and assess the situation.
- Ensure Safety: Clear the area around the person of any hazards and gently guide them to the ground if they are standing.
- Time the Seizure: Use a watch or phone to note the start and end time of the seizure. This information can be valuable for medical personnel.
- Don't Put Anything in Their Mouth: Never try to force anything into the person's mouth, including medication or food.

Part 2: Managing Seizures
Chapter 4: Responding to Seizures
4.1: Self-Management Strategies During a Seizure

- Turn on Their Side: If the person is unconscious, gently roll them onto their side to allow for easier breathing and prevent them from choking on saliva.
- Stay with Them: Stay with the person until the seizure ends and they regain consciousness.
- Call for Help: If the seizure lasts longer than 5 minutes, if the person is not breathing, or if it's their first seizure, call emergency services immediately.

Remember: Knowledge is empowering. By understanding your triggers, having a plan, and knowing how to manage a seizure, you can take control of your epilepsy and live a fulfilling life.

Part 2: Managing Seizures
Chapter 4: Responding to Seizures
4.2: Family Management Strategies During a Seizure

Witnessing a loved one experience a seizure can be a stressful and emotional event. However, by being prepared and knowing what to do, you can significantly contribute to their safety and well-being. This section provides crucial strategies for family members and caregivers to effectively manage a seizure situation.

Before a Seizure:

- Learn About Seizures: Educate yourself about different seizure types and their warning signs (auras). This knowledge allows you to anticipate and respond appropriately during a seizure.
- Develop a Seizure Action Plan: Work with your family member and their doctor to create a personalized seizure action plan. This plan should outline:
- Triggers to avoid: Identify and try to minimize exposure to known seizure triggers for your loved one.
- Actions during a seizure: This includes ensuring safety, timing the seizure, and knowing when to seek medical help.
- Post-seizure care: Plan how to comfort and support your loved one after a seizure.
- Practice Makes Perfect: Role-play seizure scenarios with your family member to become comfortable and confident in responding effectively.
- Open Communication: Maintain open communication with your loved one about their epilepsy and any concerns they might have.

Part 2: Managing Seizures
Chapter 4: Responding to Seizures
4.2: Family Management Strategies During a Seizure

During a Seizure:

- Stay Calm: It's crucial to remain calm and assess the situation. Panic can escalate the situation and hinder your ability to help effectively.

- Ensure Safety: The primary focus is ensuring your loved one's safety. Remove them from any hazards like sharp objects or hot surfaces.

- For Focal Onset Seizures: If possible, gently guide them to a safe sitting or lying position.

- For Generalized Onset Seizures: Carefully lower them to the ground to prevent injuries from falls.

- Time the Seizure: Use a watch or phone to note the start and end time of the seizure. This information can be valuable for medical personnel.

- Don't Restrain: Do not attempt to restrain the person during a seizure. This can actually cause injuries.

- Clear the Area: If possible, gently remove any objects around your loved one's face that might obstruct breathing.

- Maintain an Airway: If the person loses consciousness, gently roll them onto their side to allow for easier breathing and prevent choking on saliva.

Part 2: Managing Seizures
Chapter 4: Responding to Seizures
4.2: Family Management Strategies During a Seizure

When to Seek Medical Help:

- Seizure duration: Call emergency services if the seizure lasts longer than 5 minutes.

- Breathing difficulties: If your loved one is not breathing normally or stops breathing altogether, call for help immediately.

- First seizure: If this is the first seizure your loved one has experienced, seek medical attention to determine the cause and get appropriate treatment started.

- Concerned about recovery: If your loved one seems confused or disoriented after the seizure has ended, or if there are any injuries, call for medical evaluation.

After the Seizure:

- Offer Comfort and Support: Once the seizure subsides, stay calm and reassuring. Speak gently and offer comfort to your loved one as they regain consciousness.

- Respect Privacy: If your loved one needs time and space to recover, respect their privacy.

- Document the Seizure: If possible, briefly document details like the seizure duration, any unusual behaviors, and recovery time. This information can be helpful for future doctor visits.

Part 2: Managing Seizures
Chapter 5: Controlling Seizures
Subsection 5.1: General Treatment Considerations

Epilepsy can be a challenging condition, but with proper treatment, many people with epilepsy can live fulfilling lives. This section delves into the various treatment options available, emphasizing the importance of consulting a doctor to determine the best approach for your specific situation.

The Importance of Consulting a Doctor:

Epilepsy is a complex neurological condition, and treatment strategies need to be individualized. There's no one-size-fits-all approach. Consulting a doctor with expertise in epilepsy is crucial for:

- Accurate Diagnosis: A proper diagnosis is essential for determining the most effective treatment plan. Your doctor will consider your seizure type(s), frequency, and underlying cause (if known) to personalize your treatment approach.

- Tailored Treatment: There are various treatment options available, and your doctor will recommend the one most likely to be successful for your specific case.

- Monitoring and Adjustment: Epilepsy treatment is often an ongoing process. Your doctor will monitor your response to medication, adjust dosages as needed, and potentially explore alternative approaches if necessary.

Part 2: Managing Seizures
Chapter 5: Controlling Seizures
Subsection 5.1: General Treatment Considerations

Conventional Treatment Options:

While there are emerging treatment options on the horizon, here's an overview of some conventional approaches commonly used to manage epilepsy:

- **Antiepileptic Drugs (AEDs):** These medications are the mainstay of epilepsy treatment. They work by altering brain chemistry to prevent seizures from occurring. There are many different types of AEDs, each with its own mechanism of action and side effect profile. Your doctor will carefully select the medication(s) most appropriate for you.

- **Surgery:** In some cases, surgery may be an option, particularly for people with focal onset seizures originating from a well-defined area of the brain. Surgery aims to remove or disconnect the part of the brain causing the seizures. This is a complex decision, and a thorough evaluation by a team of specialists is necessary to determine if you're a candidate for surgery.

- **Vagal Nerve Stimulation (VNS):** This therapy involves implanting a device that sends electrical signals to the vagus nerve in the neck. These signals can help regulate brain activity and reduce seizure frequency.

Part 2: Managing Seizures
Chapter 5: Controlling Seizures
5.1: General Treatment Considerations

- **Dietary Therapies:** In some cases, specific diets, such as the ketogenic diet, may be helpful in managing seizures, particularly in children. However, these diets require careful monitoring and should only be implemented under the guidance of a healthcare professional.

It's important to note that this is not an exhaustive list of all treatment options. New therapies are constantly being developed.

Part 2: Managing Seizures
Chapter 5: Controlling Seizures
5.2: The Role of Nutrition in Epilepsy

While medications are often the mainstay of treatment for epilepsy, what you eat can also play a significant role in managing your condition. This section explores the link between nutrition and epilepsy, emphasizing the importance of consulting a registered dietitian or healthcare professional for personalized guidance.

Diet and Seizure Control:

Studies have shown that certain dietary approaches may be beneficial for some people with epilepsy, particularly children. Here's a closer look:

- **Ketogenic Diet:** This high-fat, low-carbohydrate diet forces the body to use fat for energy instead of glucose (sugar). This metabolic shift can potentially reduce seizure frequency in some individuals. However, the ketogenic diet is complex and requires careful monitoring by a healthcare professional or registered dietitian to ensure it meets your nutritional needs and is safe for long-term use.

- **Modified Atkins Diet (MAD):** This diet is a less restrictive version of the ketogenic diet, offering more flexibility in carbohydrate intake. Similar to the ketogenic diet, it should be implemented and monitored by a healthcare professional or registered dietitian.

Part 2: Managing Seizures
Chapter 5: Controlling Seizures
5.2: The Role of Nutrition in Epilepsy

Consulting a Registered Dietitian:

- **Individualized Plans**: A registered dietitian (RD) can create a personalized dietary plan that considers your specific needs, preferences, and medical history. They can help you determine if a specific dietary approach is suitable for you and guide you on safe implementation.

- **Nutritional Adequacy**: Following a restrictive diet can pose the risk of nutritional deficiencies. An RD can ensure your diet provides all the essential nutrients your body needs while managing your epilepsy.

- **Long-Term Sustainability**: Creating sustainable dietary changes is crucial for success. An RD can help you develop healthy eating habits that you can maintain for the long term.

Part 2: Managing Seizures
Chapter 5: Controlling Seizures
5.2: The Role of Nutrition in Epilepsy

Important Considerations:

- **Not a Cure:** Dietary therapies are not a cure for epilepsy, but they may be a valuable tool to complement your medication and improve seizure control.

- **Consult Your Doctor:** It's crucial to discuss any dietary changes with your doctor first. They can assess if a specific approach is suitable for you and ensure it doesn't interfere with your current medications.

- **Not for Everyone:** Dietary therapies may not be effective for everyone with epilepsy. It's important to find what works best for you in consultation with your healthcare team.

Remember: A balanced and nutritious diet is essential for overall health and well-being, and it can also play a supportive role in managing epilepsy. By consulting a registered dietitian and working with your doctor, you can explore dietary approaches safely and effectively.

Part 3: Natural and Complementary Approaches

Chapter 6: Natural Therapies for Epilepsy

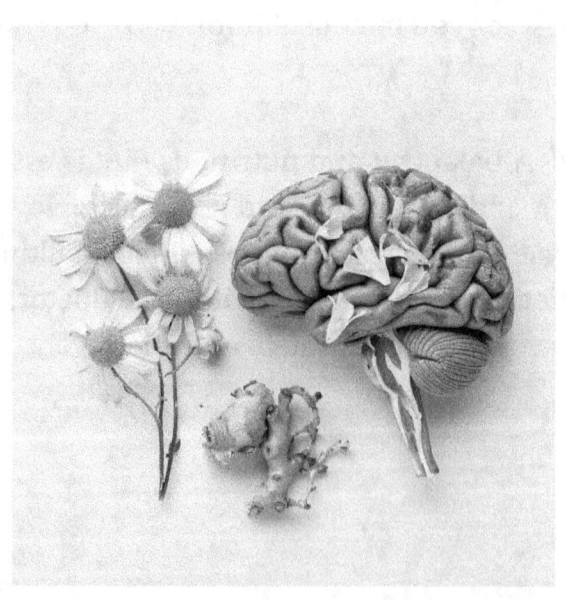

Part 3: Natural and Complementary Approaches
Chapter 6: Natural Therapies for Epilepsy

Epilepsy is a complex condition and while some natural therapies have been explored, it's important to understand that there's currently no scientific evidence to support their use as a replacement for conventional treatments. Here's a breakdown of some natural approaches and why consulting a doctor is crucial:

Natural Approaches:

- **Dietary Changes:** Certain dietary approaches, like the ketogenic diet, have shown promise in managing seizures, particularly in children. However, these diets require careful monitoring by a healthcare professional or registered dietitian to ensure safety and meet nutritional needs.

- **Herbal Remedies:** Some people with epilepsy explore herbal remedies like chamomile or valerian. However, there's a lack of conclusive evidence on their effectiveness for seizure control, and they can potentially interact with medications you're already taking.

- **Supplements:** Certain vitamins or supplements, like vitamin B6 or magnesium, have been explored for epilepsy. While some studies suggest potential benefits, more research is needed.

- **Stress Management Techniques:** Stress can be a trigger for seizures in some people. Relaxation techniques like yoga or meditation may be helpful in managing stress, but they shouldn't be used as a sole treatment for epilepsy.

Part 3: Natural and Complementary Approaches
Chapter 6: Natural Therapies for Epilepsy

Why Consulting a Doctor is Crucial:

- Safety Concerns: Some natural therapies can have side effects or interact with medications you're taking. Consulting a doctor ensures the safety and appropriateness of any natural remedy you consider.

- Potential Ineffectiveness: Natural therapies haven't been proven effective for everyone with epilepsy. A doctor can assess if a particular approach might be suitable for you as a complement to conventional treatment.

- Focus on Evidence-Based Practices: Epilepsy treatment should be grounded in scientific evidence. Your doctor can create a personalized treatment plan based on well-established practices for optimal seizure control and overall health.

Part 3: Natural and Complementary Approaches
Chapter 6: Natural Therapies for Epilepsy

Additional Considerations:

- Never Discontinue Medication: It's crucial to never stop taking your prescribed medications without consulting your doctor. Abruptly stopping medication can increase seizure risk.

- Open Communication: Maintain open communication with your doctor about any natural therapies you're considering. They can provide guidance and ensure your safety.

Remember: Epilepsy management requires a comprehensive approach. While some natural therapies might seem appealing, it's important to prioritize evidence-based treatments and consult a doctor before considering any alternative approaches. Working with your doctor, you can develop a safe and effective treatment plan that optimizes your health and well-being.

Part 3: Natural and Complementary Approaches
Chapter 6: Natural Therapies for Epilepsy
6.1: Importance of Evidence-Based Practices

Epilepsy is a complex condition, and with the vast amount of information available, it can be overwhelming to navigate treatment options. This section emphasizes the importance of evidence-based practices in managing epilepsy and underscores the crucial role of consulting a doctor to develop a personalized treatment plan.

Why Evidence-Based Practices Matter:

- Effective Treatment: Evidence-based practices are grounded in scientific research and clinical trials. This rigorous evaluation process helps ensure that the recommended treatments are actually effective in managing epilepsy and improving seizure control.

- Reduced Risk: Following evidence-based practices helps minimize the risk of trying ineffective or potentially harmful treatments.

- Improved Outcomes: By adhering to well-established treatment protocols, you increase the chances of achieving better seizure control and a higher quality of life.

Part 3: Natural and Complementary Approaches
Chapter 6: Natural Therapies for Epilepsy
6.1: Importance of Evidence-Based Practices

The Role of Your Doctor:

While this section has explored various treatment options, it's important to remember that there's no one-size-fits-all approach to epilepsy management. Consulting a doctor with expertise in epilepsy is paramount for several reasons:

- Individualized Assessment: Your doctor will consider your specific case, including seizure type(s), frequency, underlying cause (if known), age, and overall health. This personalized assessment allows them to tailor a treatment plan that addresses your unique needs.

- Weighing Risks and Benefits: Each treatment option has its own set of benefits and potential side effects. Your doctor will carefully weigh these factors to determine the most appropriate approach for you.

- Monitoring and Adjustment: Epilepsy treatment is often an ongoing process. Your doctor will monitor your response to medication, adjust dosages as needed, and explore alternative approaches if necessary. They can also address any side effects you might experience and ensure the treatment plan remains safe and effective over time.

- Emerging Therapies: The field of epilepsy treatment is constantly evolving. Your doctor can stay updated on the latest research and emerging therapies, keeping you informed about potential future options that might be suitable for you.

Part 3: Natural and Complementary Approaches
Chapter 6: Natural Therapies for Epilepsy
6.1: Importance of Evidence-Based Practices

Remember: Consulting a doctor is the best first step towards effectively managing your epilepsy. They can guide you through the maze of treatment options, ensuring you receive evidence-based care that optimizes your health and well-being.

Part 3: Natural and Complementary Approaches
Chapter 7: Exploring Specific Natural Approaches
7.1: Herbal Remedies for Epilepsy (safety and research focus)

While it's important to be aware that herbal remedies lack conclusive scientific evidence for epilepsy, here are some examples that are commonly explored, though with significant caution:

- **Chamomile:** There's limited evidence regarding chamomile's effectiveness for seizures. It might even interact with certain medications, potentially increasing seizure risk.

- **Valerian Root:** Similar to chamomile, valerian root has inconclusive research on epilepsy and may interact with medications.

- **St. John's Wort:** This herb can interact with numerous medications, including those used for epilepsy. It can also worsen seizure activity.

Important Note:

This list is not exhaustive, and there are many other herbal remedies people with epilepsy might consider.
It's crucial to reiterate that before trying any herbal remedy, consulting a doctor is essential to discuss potential risks and interactions with your current medications.

Part 3: Natural and Complementary Approaches
Chapter 7: Exploring Specific Natural Approaches
7.1: Herbal Remedies for Epilepsy (safety and research focus)

Remember:

- Safety should be your top priority. There's a lack of strong scientific evidence for most herbal remedies in treating epilepsy.

- Conventional treatment options, like medications and surgery (in specific cases), have undergone rigorous testing and are proven to be effective for seizure control.

- Focus on evidence-based practices alongside a qualified doctor to manage your epilepsy effectively.

Examples with Specific Cautions:

- **Kava:** While sometimes used for anxiety, kava can cause liver damage and shouldn't be used with certain medications, potentially worsening seizures.

- **Passionflower:** Limited research exists for passionflower and epilepsy. It might have sedative effects that could interact with medications.

- **Ginkgo** Biloba: Ginkgo biloba can increase bleeding risk and may interact with medications for epilepsy or other conditions.

Part 3: Natural and Complementary Approaches
Chapter 7: Exploring Specific Natural Approaches
7.1: Herbal Remedies for Epilepsy (safety and research focus)

General Cautions for Many Herbal Remedies:

- **Quality Variations:** Herbal remedies are often not standardized, meaning the amount of active ingredients can vary significantly between products. This makes it difficult to determine proper dosage and potential side effects.

- **Long-Term Effects:** The long-term effects of many herbal remedies are not well-understood, especially when used for chronic conditions like epilepsy.

- **Pregnancy and Breastfeeding:** Some herbal remedies can be unsafe during pregnancy or breastfeeding. It's crucial to consult a doctor before using any herbal remedy if you're pregnant or breastfeeding.

Part 3: Natural and Complementary Approaches
Chapter 7: Exploring Specific Natural Approaches
7.1: Herbal Remedies for Epilepsy (safety and research focus)

While some people with epilepsy explore herbal remedies to manage their seizures, it's crucial to emphasize safety and a lack of conclusive scientific evidence to support their use. Here's a breakdown of the key points:

Safety Concerns:

- **Limited Regulation:** Herbal remedies are often not regulated by the FDA to the same extent as prescription medications. This means their quality, purity, and potential side effects may not be well-understood.

- **Interactions with Medications:** Herbal remedies can interact with medications you're already taking for epilepsy or other conditions. These interactions can be dangerous and potentially worsen seizures.

- **Unproven Effectiveness:** There's a general lack of robust scientific research to support the effectiveness of most herbal remedies for epilepsy. They may not provide any benefit in controlling seizures.

Part 3: Natural and Complementary Approaches
Chapter 7: Exploring Specific Natural Approaches
7.1: Herbal Remedies for Epilepsy (safety and research focus)

Importance of Consulting a Doctor:

- **Safety Assessment**: A doctor can assess the potential risks and interactions of any herbal remedy you consider, helping you avoid harmful side effects.

- **Individualized Treatment**: They can develop a personalized treatment plan based on well-established practices for optimal seizure control. This may include medications, surgery (in specific cases), or dietary adjustments, depending on your individual needs.

- **Alternative Approaches**: If you're interested in exploring alternative or complementary therapies alongside conventional treatment, your doctor can guide you towards safe and potentially beneficial options like stress management techniques.

Part 3: Natural and Complementary Approaches
Chapter 7: Exploring Specific Natural Approaches
7.1: Herbal Remedies for Epilepsy (safety and research focus)

Current Research Landscape:

- **Limited Research:** While some preliminary studies have explored the effects of certain herbs on epilepsy, these studies are often small-scale and lack strong evidence. More rigorous research is needed to determine the safety and efficacy of herbal remedies for this condition.

- **Focus on Conventional Treatments:** The current focus of epilepsy research is on developing new and improved medications, surgical techniques, and other evidence-based approaches to achieve better seizure control and improve quality of life for individuals with epilepsy.

Remember:

- **Don't Discontinue Medication:** Never stop taking your prescribed medications without consulting a doctor. Abruptly stopping medication can increase seizure risk.

- **Open Communication:** Maintain open communication with your doctor about any herbal remedies you're considering. They can provide guidance based on your specific situation and medical history.

For reliable information about epilepsy treatment options, consult with a doctor or healthcare professional. They can help you create a safe and effective treatment plan that addresses your individual needs.

Part 3: Natural and Complementary Approaches
Chapter 7: Exploring Specific Natural Approaches
7.2: Vitamin Supplementation

While some people with epilepsy explore vitamin supplementation to manage their condition, the research landscape is complex. This section delves into the current understanding of vitamins and epilepsy, emphasizing the importance of consulting a doctor before taking any supplements.

Potential Benefits:

- **Addressing Deficiencies:** Certain anti-epileptic drugs (AEDs) can deplete the body's vitamin stores. In some cases, vitamin supplementation may be necessary to address these deficiencies and maintain overall health. For instance, some studies suggest that vitamin B6 deficiency might be a concern for people on long-term phenytoin use.

- **Theoretical Advantages:** Some vitamins, like vitamin D, play a role in brain function and may theoretically influence seizure activity. However, strong scientific evidence to support their direct impact on seizure control is lacking.

Part 3: Natural and Complementary Approaches
Chapter 7: Exploring Specific Natural Approaches
7.2: Vitamin Supplementation

Important Considerations:

- **Limited Evidence:** While some preliminary studies suggest potential benefits for certain vitamins, most research lacks strong evidence to definitively recommend supplementation for routine epilepsy management.

- **Focus on AEDs:** Medications are the mainstay of epilepsy treatment, and well-established AEDs have proven effective in controlling seizures. Supplementation should not be seen as a replacement for prescribed medications.

- **Potential Risks:** Taking high doses of certain vitamins can be harmful and even worsen seizures. For instance, excessive vitamin B6 intake can cause nerve damage.

The Role of Your Doctor:

- **Assessing Deficiencies:** A doctor can perform blood tests to assess your vitamin levels and determine if supplementation is necessary to address any deficiencies caused by AEDs.

- **Personalized Recommendations**: They can consider your specific needs, medical history, and current medications to determine if any vitamin supplementation is appropriate and safe for you.

Part 3: Natural and Complementary Approaches
Chapter 7: Exploring Specific Natural Approaches
7.2: Vitamin Supplementation

- **Dosage Guidance**: If supplementation is deemed necessary, your doctor will recommend the appropriate dosage to ensure you receive the benefits without potential risks.

Remember:

- **Consult a Doctor Before Supplementation:** Never take any vitamin supplements without consulting a doctor, especially if you have epilepsy and are already taking medications.

- **Focus on Evidence-Based Treatments:** Prioritize established treatment options like medications and dietary changes (in some cases) for optimal seizure control.

- **Open Communication:** Maintain open communication with your doctor about any supplements you're considering. They can provide informed guidance based on your individual situation.

Part 3: Natural and Complementary Approaches
Chapter 7: Exploring Specific Natural Approaches
7.3: Lifestyle Changes for Seizure Control (stress management, sleep hygiene, exercise)

Epilepsy management extends beyond medication. While medications are often the cornerstone of treatment, incorporating healthy lifestyle changes can significantly contribute to seizure control and improve your overall well-being. This section explores three key areas: stress management, sleep hygiene, and exercise.

1. Stress Management:

Stress can be a trigger for seizures in some people with epilepsy. By effectively managing stress, you can reduce your risk of experiencing seizures. Here are some helpful strategies:

- Relaxation Techniques: Explore relaxation techniques like yoga, meditation, or deep breathing exercises. These practices can help calm the mind and body, promoting a sense of peace and reducing stress levels.
- Cognitive Behavioral Therapy (CBT): CBT can help you identify and challenge negative thought patterns that contribute to stress. A therapist can guide you through CBT techniques to develop healthier coping mechanisms for managing stressful situations.
- Healthy Social Connections: Maintain strong social connections with supportive family and friends. Talking to loved ones about your worries and experiences can be a powerful stress reliever.

Part 3: Natural and Complementary Approaches
Chapter 7: Exploring Specific Natural Approaches
7.3: Lifestyle Changes for Seizure Control (stress management, sleep hygiene, exercise)

2. Sleep Hygiene:

Sleep deprivation is another known trigger for seizures. Prioritizing good sleep hygiene can significantly improve your sleep quality and potentially reduce seizure risk. Here are some tips:

- **Establish a Regular Sleep Schedule**: Go to bed and wake up at consistent times each day, even on weekends. This helps regulate your body's natural sleep-wake cycle.

- **Create a Relaxing Bedtime Routine**: Develop a calming bedtime routine that signals to your body it's time to wind down. This could include taking a warm bath, reading a book, or practicing relaxation techniques.

- **Optimize Your Sleep Environment**: Ensure your bedroom is dark, quiet, and cool. Invest in blackout curtains, earplugs, and a comfortable mattress to promote better sleep quality.

Part 3: Natural and Complementary Approaches
Chapter 7: Exploring Specific Natural Approaches
7.3: Lifestyle Changes for Seizure Control (stress management, sleep hygiene, exercise)

3. Exercise:

Regular physical activity offers numerous health benefits, including improved mood, stress reduction, and better sleep. These factors can all contribute to seizure control. Here are some exercise considerations:

- **Choose Activities You Enjoy:** Find physical activities you enjoy, such as walking, swimming, cycling, or dancing. This makes it more likely you'll stick with an exercise routine.
- **Start Gradually:** If you're new to exercise, begin slowly and gradually increase the duration and intensity of your workouts as your fitness improves.
- **Maintain Consistency:** Aim for at least 30 minutes of moderate-intensity exercise most days of the week. Consistency is key to reaping the long-term benefits of exercise.

Important Considerations:

- Consult Your Doctor: Before starting any new exercise program, consult your doctor to ensure it's safe for you, especially if you have any limitations or health concerns.

- Plan Around Seizures: If you experience frequent seizures, discuss strategies with your doctor to manage your exercise routine safely. This might involve exercising with a partner or in safe environments.

Part 3: Natural and Complementary Approaches
Chapter 7: Exploring Specific Natural Approaches
7.3: Lifestyle Changes for Seizure Control (stress management, sleep hygiene, exercise)

Remember: Lifestyle changes take time and effort, but incorporating these practices into your daily routine can significantly improve your overall health and potentially contribute to better seizure control. By working with your doctor and adopting healthy habits, you can take charge of your epilepsy and live a fulfilling life.

Part 3: Natural and Complementary Approaches
Chapter 8: Alternative Therapies for Epilepsy

The term "alternative therapies" can be misleading for epilepsy management. Epilepsy is a complex neurological condition, and evidence-based medical treatments should be the foundation of your treatment plan. These include medications, dietary changes (in some cases), and surgery (for specific situations).

However, some people with epilepsy explore complementary therapies alongside conventional treatment. Here's a breakdown of this approach, with a strong emphasis on consulting a doctor first:

Complementary Therapies:

- **Focus:** These therapies aim to complement your main treatment plan, potentially improving your overall well-being and potentially reducing seizure frequency.

- **Examples:** Stress management techniques (yoga, meditation), relaxation techniques, sleep hygiene practices, and certain dietary approaches (under medical supervision).

Part 3: Natural and Complementary Approaches
Chapter 8: Alternative Therapies for Epilepsy

Why Consulting a Doctor is Crucial:

- **Safety:** Some complementary therapies, like herbal remedies, can have side effects or interact with medications you're taking. A doctor can assess the safety of any complementary therapy you consider.

- **Focus on Evidence-Based Practices:** A doctor can ensure your treatment plan prioritizes medications, surgery (if applicable), or dietary adjustments with proven effectiveness for seizure control.

- **Individualized Approach:** They can consider your specific needs, medical history, and current medications to determine if any complementary therapy might be suitable for you.

Important Considerations:

- **Limited Evidence:** Many complementary therapies lack strong scientific evidence to support their direct impact on seizure control.

- **Not a Replacement:** Complementary therapies should never be used as a replacement for conventional epilepsy treatment.

- **Open Communication:** Maintain open communication with your doctor about any complementary therapies you're interested in exploring.

Part 3: Natural and Complementary Approaches
Chapter 8: Alternative Therapies for Epilepsy

Here are some additional points to remember:

- Never Discontinue Medication: Always consult your doctor before stopping any prescribed medications.

- Focus on Safety: Avoid any complementary therapies that haven't been discussed with your doctor and cleared for safety.

- Reliable Sources: If you're researching complementary therapies, seek information from reputable sources like the National Institutes of Health (NIH) or epilepsy organizations.

Remember: The safest and most effective way to manage epilepsy is to work with a qualified healthcare professional. They can develop a personalized treatment plan based on well-researched and proven approaches, while also considering your interest in exploring complementary therapies for potential benefits.

Part 3: Natural and Complementary Approaches
Chapter 8: Alternative Therapies for Epilepsy
8.1: Acupuncture

Acupuncture is a traditional Chinese medicine practice involving inserting thin needles into specific points on the body. While some people with epilepsy explore acupuncture for seizure control, the research landscape is complex. Here's a breakdown of what we currently know:

Potential Benefits:

- Limited Research: Some studies suggest acupuncture might be helpful in reducing seizure frequency, although the evidence is not conclusive.
- Complementary Approach: Acupuncture may be seen as a complementary therapy alongside conventional epilepsy treatment, potentially improving overall well-being and possibly reducing seizure frequency.

Important Considerations:

- Lack of Strong Evidence: More robust research is needed to definitively determine the effectiveness of acupuncture for epilepsy.
- Focus on Established Treatments: Medications, dietary changes (in specific cases), and surgery (for specific situations) are well-established and proven effective for seizure control. Acupuncture should not be considered a replacement.
- Potential Risks: While generally safe with qualified practitioners, minor side effects like soreness or bleeding at the insertion points can occur. There's also a small risk of infection if sterile needles aren't used.

Part 3: Natural and Complementary Approaches
Chapter 8: Alternative Therapies for Epilepsy
8.1: Acupuncture

The Role of Your Doctor:

- Assessment: A doctor can assess if you're a good candidate for acupuncture, considering your medical history and current medications.
- Treatment Plan: They can ensure acupuncture complements your established treatment plan and doesn't interfere with medication effectiveness.
- Referral: If you decide to explore acupuncture, your doctor can refer you to a qualified and licensed acupuncturist.

Remember:

- Consult a Doctor Before Trying Acupuncture: Never start acupuncture without your doctor's knowledge and approval.
- Focus on Evidence-Based Treatments: Prioritize established approaches like medication and dietary changes for optimal seizure control.
- Open Communication: Maintain open communication with your doctor about your interest in acupuncture. They can guide you based on your individual situation.

Part 3: Natural and Complementary Approaches
Chapter 8: Alternative Therapies for Epilepsy
8.2: Massage

Massage therapy is a technique involving applying pressure to the muscles and soft tissues of the body. While there's no definitive evidence that massage directly controls seizures, it can offer some potential benefits for people with epilepsy. Here's a closer look:

Potential Benefits:

- Stress Reduction: Massage can promote relaxation and reduce stress, which may be a seizure trigger for some people with epilepsy. By lowering stress levels, massage therapy might create a more calming environment and potentially reduce seizure frequency.

- Improved Sleep Quality: Massage can also promote better sleep, another factor that can influence seizure control. Improved sleep hygiene can contribute to overall well-being and potentially reduce seizure risk.

- Pain Management: If you experience muscle tension or pain related to epilepsy or its treatment, massage therapy may offer some relief.

Part 3: Natural and Complementary Approaches
Chapter 8: Alternative Therapies for Epilepsy
8.2: Massage

Important Considerations:

- Limited Research: There's a lack of strong scientific evidence to definitively prove that massage directly reduces seizure frequency.

- Focus on Conventional Treatments: Medications, dietary changes (in some cases), and surgery (for specific situations) are well-established and proven effective for seizure control. Massage should not be considered a replacement.

- Communication with Doctor: Before starting massage therapy, discuss it with your doctor. They can advise on whether it's suitable for you and ensure it complements your existing treatment plan.

Types of Massage to Consider:

- Swedish Massage: This is a gentle and relaxing form of massage that focuses on promoting relaxation and improving circulation.

- Chair Massage: This is a shorter massage done while you're seated in a special chair. It can be a good option if you have mobility limitations.

Part 3: Natural and Complementary Approaches
Chapter 8: Alternative Therapies for Epilepsy
8.2: Massage

Cautions and Considerations:

- Certain Techniques: Avoid massage techniques that involve forceful manipulation or deep pressure on the head or neck, as these might theoretically trigger seizures in some people.

- Communicate with Therapist: Inform your massage therapist about your epilepsy and any specific concerns you might have.

- Start Gently: Begin with a short massage session and see how you feel before booking longer sessions.

Remember:

- Consult Your Doctor First: Always discuss massage therapy with your doctor before starting it.
- Focus on Evidence-Based Treatments: Prioritize established treatments like medications and dietary changes for optimal seizure control.
- Open Communication: Maintain open communication with your doctor about your interest in massage therapy. They can guide you based on your individual situation.
- By working with your doctor and choosing appropriate massage techniques, you can explore the potential benefits of massage therapy for relaxation and potentially improve your overall well-being while managing your epilepsy.

Part 3: Natural and Complementary Approaches
Chapter 8: Alternative Therapies for Epilepsy
8.3: Mind-Body Approaches (meditation, yoga)

Epilepsy management goes beyond medication. Mind-body approaches like meditation and yoga have gained increasing interest for their potential to complement conventional treatment and improve overall well-being in people with epilepsy. Here's a breakdown of these practices and why consulting a doctor is crucial.

Benefits of Mind-Body Approaches:

- Stress Reduction: Stress can be a trigger for seizures in some individuals. Techniques like meditation and yoga promote relaxation, potentially reducing stress levels and lowering seizure risk.
- Improved Sleep Quality: Both practices can also contribute to better sleep, another factor that can influence seizure control. Adequate sleep hygiene is crucial for overall health and may indirectly reduce seizure risk.
- Enhanced Self-Awareness: Mind-body approaches can cultivate greater self-awareness, allowing you to identify early warning signs (auras) of potential seizures and take appropriate measures.
- Improved Coping Mechanisms: These practices can equip you with better tools to manage stress and anxiety, which can be beneficial for overall well-being and potentially reduce seizure frequency.

Part 3: Natural and Complementary Approaches
Chapter 8: Alternative Therapies for Epilepsy
8.3: Mind-Body Approaches (meditation, yoga)

Types of Mind-Body Approaches:

- **Meditation**: Meditation involves focusing your attention and quieting the mind. There are various meditation techniques, such as mindfulness meditation, which can be practiced anywhere.

- **Yoga**: Yoga combines physical postures, breathing exercises, and meditation. Certain yoga styles may be better suited for people with epilepsy than others.

Why Consulting a Doctor is Important:

- Safety: A doctor can assess if you're a good candidate for these practices, considering your seizure type, frequency, and any physical limitations. They can also advise on modifications to poses or exercises if needed.
- Complementary Approach: Your doctor can ensure mind-body techniques complement your established treatment plan and don't interfere with medication effectiveness.
- Finding the Right Fit: They may be able to recommend classes or resources tailored to people with epilepsy or can guide you in finding a qualified instructor who understands your condition.

Part 3: Natural and Complementary Approaches
Chapter 8: Alternative Therapies for Epilepsy
8.3: Mind-Body Approaches (meditation, yoga)

Additional Considerations:

- Research is Ongoing: While studies suggest potential benefits, more research is warranted to definitively determine the impact of mind-body approaches on seizure control.

- Focus on Evidence-Based Treatments: Medications, dietary changes (in specific cases), and surgery (for specific situations) remain the cornerstone of epilepsy treatment.

- Open Communication: Maintain open communication with your doctor about your interest in mind-body approaches. They can guide you based on your individual situation.

Here are some resources to get you started:

- National Center for Complementary and Integrative Health (NCCIH): https://www.ncbi.nlm.nih.gov/pmc/articles/PMC6413605/
- Epilepsy Foundation: https://www.epilepsy.com/stories/helping-epilepsy-patients-yoga

Part 3: Natural and Complementary Approaches
Chapter 8: Alternative Therapies for Epilepsy
8.3: Mind-Body Approaches (meditation, yoga)

Remember: Mind-body approaches can be a valuable addition to your epilepsy management plan, but they should not replace conventional treatment options. By working with your doctor and finding practices that suit you, you can explore the potential benefits of mind-body approaches for relaxation, improved well-being, and potentially reduced seizure frequency.

Part 4: Living Well with Epilepsy

Chapter 9: Importance of Sleep (combines "Sleep and Epilepsy")

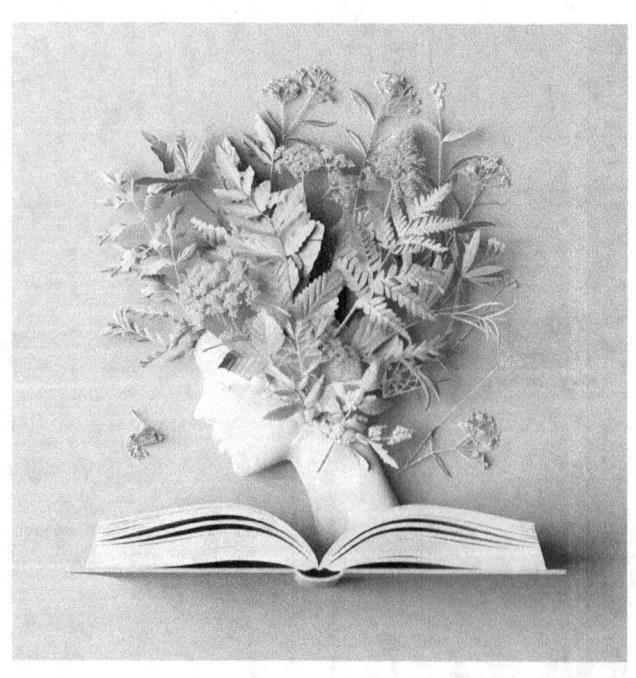

Part 4: Living Well with Epilepsy
Chapter 9: Importance of Sleep (combines "Sleep and Epilepsy")

Sleep and epilepsy are intricately linked. Disrupted sleep patterns can worsen seizures, and conversely, seizures themselves can fragment sleep. This section explores the importance of sleep for epilepsy management and emphasizes healthy sleep hygiene practices.

Sleep's Impact on Epilepsy:

- Seizure Trigger: Sleep deprivation is a well-known trigger for seizures in many people with epilepsy. Not getting enough quality sleep can lower the seizure threshold, making them more likely to occur.

- Seizure Disruption: Seizures themselves can disrupt sleep architecture. After a seizure, you might experience difficulty falling asleep, staying asleep, or experience fragmented sleep with frequent awakenings. This can worsen sleep quality and perpetuate a cycle of sleep deprivation and seizures.

Part 4: Living Well with Epilepsy
Chapter 9: Importance of Sleep (combines "Sleep and Epilepsy")

Prioritizing Healthy Sleep:

- Regular Sleep Schedule: Establish a consistent sleep schedule, going to bed and waking up at roughly the same time each day, even on weekends. This helps regulate your body's natural sleep-wake cycle.

- Relaxing Bedtime Routine: Develop a calming bedtime routine that signals to your body it's time to wind down. This could include taking a warm bath, reading a book, or practicing relaxation techniques like meditation.

- Optimize Your Sleep Environment: Ensure your bedroom is dark, quiet, and cool. Invest in blackout curtains, earplugs, and a comfortable mattress to promote better sleep quality.

- Limit Screen Time Before Bed: The blue light emitted from electronic devices can suppress melatonin production, a hormone that regulates sleep. Avoid screens for at least an hour before bedtime.

- Regular Exercise: Regular physical activity can improve sleep quality. However, avoid strenuous exercise close to bedtime, as it can be stimulating.

Part 4: Living Well with Epilepsy
Chapter 9: Importance of Sleep (combines "Sleep and Epilepsy")

Additional Tips:

- Manage Stress: Stress can worsen both sleep and seizures. Techniques like yoga, meditation, or deep breathing exercises can help reduce stress and promote relaxation.
- Avoid Caffeine and Alcohol: Limit caffeine intake, especially in the afternoon and evening, as it can interfere with sleep. Avoid alcohol close to bedtime, as it can disrupt sleep architecture.
- See a Doctor for Sleep Problems: If you continue to experience sleep problems despite implementing healthy sleep hygiene practices, consult your doctor. They can rule out any underlying sleep disorders and recommend additional strategies.

Remember: Prioritizing good sleep hygiene is crucial for managing epilepsy. By getting enough quality sleep, you can potentially reduce your risk of seizures and improve your overall health and well-being. Working with your doctor, you can develop a personalized sleep plan to optimize your sleep quality and support your epilepsy management effectively.

This section builds upon the information previously covered in "Nighttime Seizures" by emphasizing the importance of sleep hygiene practices for overall seizure control.

Part 4: Living Well with Epilepsy
Chapter 10: Understanding Seizure Effects

Seizures can manifest in a variety of ways, and the effects can vary depending on the type, location, and duration of the seizure. Here's a breakdown of some potential seizure effects:

Physical Effects:

- Muscle Stiffness or Jerking: This is a common symptom, particularly in tonic-clonic seizures (formerly grand mal seizures) where the body stiffens (tonic) followed by jerking movements (clonic).

- Loss of Consciousness: Depending on the seizure type, you might lose awareness of your surroundings for a brief period.

- Sensory Disturbances: Some people experience strange smells, tastes, or visual auras before or during a seizure.

- Autonomic Symptoms: These can include changes in heart rate, breathing, sweating, or nausea.

- Urinary or Bowel Incontinence: This can occur in some seizure types, particularly during prolonged seizures.

- Injury: During a seizure, especially if you fall or strike objects, there's a risk of injury.

Part 4: Living Well with Epilepsy
Chapter 10: Understanding Seizure Effects

Cognitive and Emotional Effects:

- Confusion: After a seizure, you might experience temporary confusion and difficulty thinking clearly. This can last for minutes or even hours.

- Headache: Headaches are a common after-effect of seizures.

- Fatigue: Seizures can be physically draining and leave you feeling tired.

- Fear or Anxiety: The experience of a seizure can be frightening, and it's natural to feel anxious or worried after one occurs.

Long-Term Effects:

- Memory Problems: Frequent seizures can sometimes lead to memory problems.

- Learning Difficulties: In children, uncontrolled seizures can affect learning and development.

- Psychological Issues: People with epilepsy are more at risk for depression, anxiety, and social isolation.

Part 4: Living Well with Epilepsy
Chapter 10: Understanding Seizure Effects

Importance of Consulting a Doctor:

- Understanding Your Seizures: A doctor can help you understand your specific seizure type and the potential effects you might experience.
- Treatment Plan: They can develop a personalized treatment plan to manage your seizures and minimize their effects.
- Addressing Concerns: Discuss any concerns you have about seizure effects with your doctor. They can provide guidance and support.

Remember: Experiencing seizures can be physically and emotionally challenging. However, with proper treatment and support, you can manage your epilepsy and live a fulfilling life.

Part 4: Living Well with Epilepsy
Chapter 10: Understanding Seizure Effects
10.1: Breathing and Autonomic Disturbances

Seizures can disrupt the autonomic nervous system, which controls involuntary functions like breathing, heart rate, blood pressure, and digestion. Here's a closer look at how seizures can affect breathing and some potential autonomic disturbances:

Breathing Problems During Seizures:

- Apnea: This is a temporary cessation of breathing, which can occur during some seizure types. It can be a life-threatening complication if it lasts for a prolonged period.

- Irregular Breathing: Seizures can cause changes in breathing patterns, making breathing shallow, rapid, or labored.

Factors Affecting Breathing:

- Seizure Type: The type, location, and severity of the seizure can influence the likelihood and severity of breathing problems.

- Brain Region Involved: Seizures involving the brainstem, which controls breathing, are more likely to cause respiratory issues.

Part 4: Living Well with Epilepsy
Chapter 10: Understanding Seizure Effects
10.1: Breathing and Autonomic Disturbances

Autonomic Disturbances:

- Cardiovascular: Seizures can cause changes in heart rate and blood pressure. Some people might experience tachycardia (fast heart rate) or bradycardia (slow heart rate) during or after a seizure.

- Gastrointestinal: Seizures can trigger nausea, vomiting, or abdominal discomfort.

- Urinary and Bowel Incontinence: Loss of bladder or bowel control can occur during prolonged seizures.

Importance of Monitoring:

- Awareness: Being aware of potential breathing difficulties and autonomic disturbances is crucial for both people with epilepsy and their caregivers.

- Monitoring: During or after a seizure, monitor breathing patterns and be alert for signs of respiratory distress like gasping or blueish skin discoloration (cyanosis).

- Seek Help: If breathing difficulties occur or don't resolve promptly after a seizure, call emergency services immediately.

Part 4: Living Well with Epilepsy
Chapter 10: Understanding Seizure Effects
10.1: Breathing and Autonomic Disturbances

Additional Considerations:

- Post-Seizure State: Confusion and drowsiness after a seizure can make it difficult to communicate potential breathing problems.
- SUDEP (Sudden Unexpected Death in Epilepsy): In rare cases, breathing difficulties during a seizure can contribute to SUDEP.
- If you have concerns about breathing problems or autonomic disturbances during seizures, discuss them with your doctor. They can assess your individual risk factors and provide guidance on monitoring and safety measures.

Here are some additional resources:

- National Institute of Neurological Disorders and Stroke: https://www.ninds.nih.gov/health-information/disorders/epilepsy-and-seizures
- Epilepsy Foundation: https://www.epilcpsy.com/

Remember: Early recognition and intervention are crucial for managing breathing difficulties and autonomic disturbances during seizures. By working with your doctor and implementing safety measures, you can minimize risks and ensure optimal care during and after a seizure.

Part 4: Living Well with Epilepsy
Chapter 10: Understanding Seizure Effects
10.2: Consequences of Seizures (cognitive and other long-term effects)

Seizures can have a range of consequences, both in the short-term (during or immediately after a seizure) and long-term (lasting effects). Here's a breakdown of the potential cognitive and other long-term effects of seizures:

Cognitive Effects:

- Memory Problems: Frequent seizures, particularly those involving the temporal lobe (which plays a role in memory), can lead to memory difficulties. These might involve forgetting recent events, difficulty learning new information, or problems with short-term memory.

- Attention and Concentration: Seizures can impair your ability to focus and concentrate. You might experience difficulty following conversations, completing tasks, or staying on track mentally.

- Learning Difficulties: In children with uncontrolled seizures, cognitive issues can affect their academic performance and development.

- Slower Processing Speed: Some people with epilepsy experience a slower processing speed, meaning it takes them longer to understand and respond to information.

Part 4: Living Well with Epilepsy
Chapter 10: Understanding Seizure Effects
10.2: Consequences of Seizures (cognitive and other long-term effects)

Factors Affecting Cognitive Effects:

- Seizure Type and Frequency: The type, location, and severity of seizures, as well as their frequency, can influence the likelihood and severity of cognitive problems.
- Age of Onset: Children whose epilepsy starts at a young age are more vulnerable to cognitive difficulties.
- Underlying Cause: The underlying cause of epilepsy can also play a role in cognitive effects.

Other Long-Term Effects:

- Psychological Issues: People with epilepsy are more at risk for developing depression, anxiety, or social isolation due to the challenges of living with the condition.
- Social Stigma: In some cases, epilepsy can carry a social stigma, which can contribute to feelings of isolation and low self-esteem.
- Increased Risk of Injuries: During a seizure, there's a risk of injuries from falls or collisions with objects.
- Bone Health Issues: Certain anti-epileptic medications (AEDs) can affect bone density, increasing the risk of osteoporosis over time.

Part 4: Living Well with Epilepsy
Chapter 10: Understanding Seizure Effects
10.2: Consequences of Seizures (cognitive and other long-term effects)

Importance of Early Diagnosis and Treatment:

- Minimizing Seizure Frequency: The most crucial factor in preventing long-term effects is controlling seizure frequency with proper diagnosis and treatment.
- Addressing Cognitive Issues: If you experience cognitive difficulties, talk to your doctor. There might be interventions or cognitive rehabilitation strategies to help manage these challenges.
- Mental Health Support: Don't hesitate to seek help for mental health concerns like depression or anxiety. Support groups and therapy can be beneficial.

Remember: The long-term effects of seizures can vary greatly depending on individual circumstances. With proper treatment and management, many people with epilepsy can live fulfilling lives.

Part 4: Living Well with Epilepsy
Chapter 11: Self-Management for Epilepsy

Epilepsy management extends beyond medication. Self-management practices empower you to take an active role in your epilepsy care, potentially reducing seizure frequency and improving your overall well-being. This section combines strategies for managing seizures and coping with the emotional aspects of epilepsy.

Strategies for Seizure Control:

- Medication Adherence: Taking your medications exactly as prescribed is crucial for seizure control. Don't skip doses or adjust your medication regimen without consulting your doctor.

- Seizure Triggers: Identify and avoid your seizure triggers whenever possible. Common triggers include lack of sleep, stress, certain medications, and flashing lights.

- Keeping a Seizure Diary: Track your seizures in a diary, noting details like date, time, potential triggers, and seizure characteristics. This information can help your doctor identify patterns and adjust your treatment plan if needed.

- Healthy Lifestyle Habits: Prioritize good sleep hygiene practices, regular exercise, and a balanced diet. These habits can contribute to overall health and potentially reduce seizure risk.

Part 4: Living Well with Epilepsy
Chapter 11: Self-Management for Epilepsy

- Stress Management Techniques: Techniques like yoga, meditation, or deep breathing exercises can help reduce stress, a known trigger for seizures in some people.

- Open Communication with Doctor: Maintain open communication with your doctor about your seizures, concerns, and any self-management strategies you're considering.

Coping with Epilepsy:

- Emotional Challenges: Living with epilepsy can be emotionally challenging. Don't hesitate to seek support if you experience anxiety, depression, or feelings of isolation. Support groups, therapy, or talking to a trusted friend or family member can be helpful.

- Social Stigma: Epilepsy can carry a social stigma in some cases. Education and open communication with loved ones can help dispel myths and promote understanding.

- Maintaining a Positive Attitude: A positive outlook can significantly impact your well-being. Focus on what you can control and celebrate your achievements in managing your epilepsy.

- Finding Support: Connect with epilepsy organizations or support groups to connect with others who understand the challenges you face. This can be a source of valuable information, encouragement, and emotional support.

Part 4: Living Well with Epilepsy
Chapter 11: Self-Management for Epilepsy

Remember:

- Self-management is a journey, not a destination. It takes time and effort to find what works best for you.
- Work with your doctor. They are your partner in managing your epilepsy and can guide you in implementing effective self-management strategies.
- Focus on a holistic approach. Self-management encompasses various aspects, including medication adherence, lifestyle changes, emotional well-being, and navigating the social aspects of epilepsy.
- By taking an active role in your epilepsy care, you can empower yourself to live a fulfilling and healthy life.

Part 4: Living Well with Epilepsy
Chapter 11: Self-Management for Epilepsy
11.1: Techniques for Managing Your Condition

Epilepsy management goes beyond just medication. Here's a breakdown of various techniques you can incorporate into your routine to effectively manage your condition:

Medical Management:

- Medications: Anti-epileptic drugs (AEDs) are the cornerstone of epilepsy treatment. Taking them exactly as prescribed is crucial for seizure control. Your doctor will determine the most appropriate medication and dosage for you.

- Dietary Changes (in specific cases): In some cases, specific dietary approaches like the ketogenic diet can be helpful for managing seizures, particularly in children. However, these diets should only be implemented under strict medical supervision.

- Surgery (for specific situations): For some people with epilepsy, surgery may be an option if medications and other approaches haven't been successful.

Part 4: Living Well with Epilepsy
Chapter 11: Self-Management for Epilepsy
11.1: Techniques for Managing Your Condition

Self-Management Strategies:

- Seizure Triggers: Identifying and avoiding your seizure triggers can significantly reduce your risk of experiencing seizures. Common triggers include lack of sleep, stress, certain medications, and flashing lights.

- Seizure Diary: Keeping a seizure diary is a valuable tool. Track details like date, time, potential triggers, and seizure characteristics. This information can help your doctor identify patterns and adjust your treatment plan if needed.

- Healthy Lifestyle Habits: Prioritize good sleep hygiene practices, regular exercise, and a balanced diet. These habits promote overall health and can potentially reduce seizure risk.

- Stress Management Techniques: Stress can be a trigger for seizures in some people. Techniques like yoga, meditation, or deep breathing exercises can help manage stress.

- Medication Adherence: Always take your medications exactly as prescribed by your doctor. Skipping doses or adjusting your medication regimen on your own can worsen seizures.

Part 4: Living Well with Epilepsy
Chapter 11: Self-Management for Epilepsy
11.1: Techniques for Managing Your Condition

Complementary Therapies (consult a doctor before starting):

- Mind-Body Approaches: Techniques like meditation and yoga may promote relaxation, potentially reducing stress and lowering seizure risk. However, consult your doctor before starting any new practices to ensure they don't interfere with your medications or worsen seizures.

- Alternative Therapies: While some explore alternative therapies like acupuncture or massage, there's limited evidence for their direct impact on seizure control. Consult your doctor before trying any alternative therapy to discuss potential risks and benefits.

Coping and Emotional Wellbeing:

- Support Groups: Connecting with epilepsy organizations or support groups allows you to connect with others who understand the challenges you face. This can be a source of valuable information, encouragement, and emotional support.

- Therapy: Don't hesitate to seek professional help if you experience anxiety, depression, or feelings of isolation. Therapy can equip you with coping mechanisms to manage the emotional aspects of epilepsy.

Part 4: Living Well with Epilepsy
Chapter 11: Self-Management for Epilepsy
11.1: Techniques for Managing Your Condition

- Maintaining a Positive Attitude: A positive outlook can significantly impact your well-being. Focus on what you can control and celebrate your achievements in managing your epilepsy.

Remember:

- Individualized Approach: The most effective techniques will vary depending on your specific type of epilepsy, triggers, and overall health. Work with your doctor to develop a personalized management plan.

- Communication is Key: Maintain open communication with your doctor about your seizures, concerns, and any self-management strategies you're considering.

- Empowerment Through Knowledge: Educate yourself about epilepsy to better understand your condition and feel empowered to manage it effectively.

By incorporating these techniques into your life and working collaboratively with your doctor, you can take charge of your epilepsy and live a fulfilling life.

Part 4: Living Well with Epilepsy
Chapter 11: Self-Management for Epilepsy
11.2: Emotional and Social Support

Epilepsy can take a toll on your emotional and social well-being. This section highlights the importance of emotional and social support, explores the benefits of support groups, and emphasizes the value of addressing mental health concerns.

The Impact of Epilepsy:

- Emotional Challenges: Living with epilepsy can be emotionally challenging. You might experience anxiety, depression, frustration, or feelings of isolation. These emotions are understandable and can affect your overall well-being.

- Social Stigma: In some cases, epilepsy can carry a social stigma. People with epilepsy might face misunderstanding, discrimination, or social isolation.

The Power of Support:

- Reduced Stress and Anxiety: Having a strong support system can help reduce stress and anxiety, which can be triggers for seizures in some people.

- Improved Coping Mechanisms: Support groups and therapy can equip you with coping mechanisms to navigate the emotional challenges of living with epilepsy.

- Sense of Belonging: Connecting with others who understand your experiences can foster a sense of belonging and reduce feelings of isolation.

Part 4: Living Well with Epilepsy
Chapter 11: Self-Management for Epilepsy
11.2: Emotional and Social Support

Benefits of Support Groups:

- Shared Experiences: Support groups provide a safe space to connect with others who share your experiences. You can learn from each other, offer encouragement, and build a sense of community.

- Information Sharing: Support groups can be a valuable source of information about epilepsy management, coping strategies, and resources available in your area.

- Emotional Validation: Knowing you're not alone in facing these challenges can be incredibly validating and supportive.

Addressing Mental Health Concerns:

- Don't Hesitate to Seek Help: If you experience anxiety, depression, or social isolation, don't hesitate to seek professional help. Therapy can equip you with tools to manage these challenges and improve your overall well-being.

- Mental Health and Epilepsy: People with epilepsy are more at risk for developing mental health conditions. Open communication with your doctor can ensure you receive the support you need for both your physical and mental health.

Part 4: Living Well with Epilepsy
Chapter 11: Self-Management for Epilepsy
11.2: Emotional and Social Support

Finding Support Groups:

- Epilepsy Organizations: Many epilepsy organizations offer support groups in person or online. The Epilepsy Foundation (https://www.epilepsy.com/) is a good starting point to find resources in your area.

- Online Support Groups: Several online forums and communities offer support for people with epilepsy.

Remember:

- You're Not Alone: Many people live with epilepsy, and a strong support system can significantly improve your quality of life.

- Prioritize Your Well-being: Your emotional and mental health are crucial aspects of overall well-being. Don't hesitate to seek help if you're struggling.

- Take Charge: Building a network of support is an active process. Reach out to organizations, therapists, or online communities to find the support that works best for you.

By prioritizing emotional and social support, you can build resilience and manage the challenges of living with epilepsy. You can find strength and encouragement through connecting with others who understand and navigate your journey.

Part 5: The Future of Epilepsy Treatment

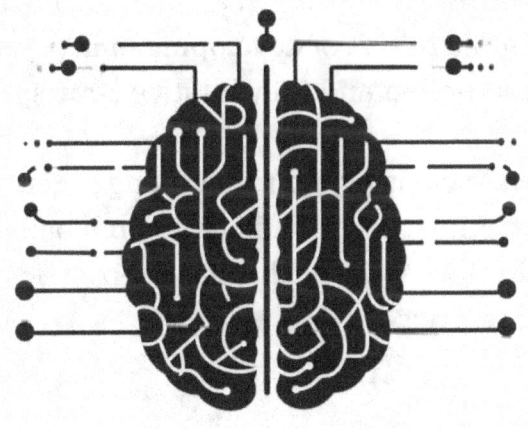

Part 5: The Future of Epilepsy Treatment

The future of epilepsy treatment is exciting and holds promise for significantly improving the lives of people with epilepsy. Here's a glimpse into some of the emerging areas of research and potential breakthroughs:

1. Improved Diagnostics and Personalized Medicine:

- Advanced Imaging Techniques: Newer brain imaging techniques like functional MRI (fMRI) and magnetoencephalography (MEG) may improve the accuracy of seizure focus localization, allowing for more targeted treatment approaches.

- Genetic Testing: Advances in genetic testing may help identify people at risk of developing epilepsy, allowing for earlier intervention and preventative strategies.

- Biomarkers: Scientists are researching potential biomarkers (measurable indicators) in blood or other bodily fluids to predict or diagnose seizures and assess treatment response.

Part 5: The Future of Epilepsy Treatment

2. Targeted and Minimally Invasive Therapies:

- Minimally Invasive Surgical Techniques: Newer, minimally invasive surgical procedures like laser ablation may offer more precise targeting of seizure foci with reduced recovery times.

- Neuromodulation Therapies: Advanced neuromodulation therapies like deep brain stimulation (DBS) and responsive neurostimulation (RNS) are being refined to offer more personalized and precise seizure control.

- Closed-Loop Systems: These are implantable devices that can detect seizure activity and deliver targeted stimulation to prevent seizures before they occur.

3. Gene Therapy and Gene Editing:

- Gene Therapy: This approach aims to deliver healthy genes to replace or repair faulty genes that contribute to epilepsy. While still in early stages, it has the potential to offer a long-term cure for some forms of epilepsy.

- Gene Editing: CRISPR-Cas9 gene editing technology has the potential to modify genes associated with epilepsy, potentially offering a permanent solution in the future.

Part 5: The Future of Epilepsy Treatment

4. Improved Medications and Drug Delivery Systems:

- Anti-Seizure Medications: Research is ongoing to develop new and more effective medications with fewer side effects.

- Targeted Drug Delivery: Scientists are exploring ways to deliver medications directly to the seizure focus in the brain, minimizing side effects on other parts of the body.

Important Considerations:

- Research is Ongoing: While these advancements are promising, most are still under investigation or in early stages of development. It may take time before they become widely available treatment options.

- Individualized Treatment: The future of epilepsy treatment is likely to move towards personalized medicine, with treatment plans tailored to the specific type and cause of epilepsy in each individual.

- Importance of Continued Research: Continued funding and research efforts are crucial to bring these potential breakthroughs to fruition and improve the lives of people with epilepsy.

Remember: The field of epilepsy treatment is constantly evolving, offering hope for a future where epilepsy can be effectively managed or even cured.

Part 5: The Future of Epilepsy Treatment
Chapter 12: Looking Ahead: Future Treatments and Technologies

Epilepsy has traditionally been a challenging condition to manage, but the future holds immense promise for improved treatments and technologies. Here's a breakdown of some exciting advancements on the horizon:

1. Enhanced Diagnostics and Personalized Medicine:

Imagine a future where epilepsy diagnosis is more precise and treatment plans are tailored to your specific needs. This future is getting closer thanks to:

- Advanced Brain Imaging: Techniques like functional MRI (fMRI) and magnetoencephalography (MEG) are becoming more sophisticated, allowing for better localization of seizure origin in the brain. This can lead to more targeted treatment approaches.

- Genetic Testing: Advances in genetic testing may help identify individuals predisposed to epilepsy, enabling earlier intervention and potentially preventing seizures altogether.

- Biomarkers: Researchers are exploring potential biomarkers in blood or other fluids that could predict seizures, diagnose epilepsy, and assess treatment response. This personalized approach would revolutionize epilepsy management.

Part 5: The Future of Epilepsy Treatment
Chapter 12: Looking Ahead: Future Treatments and Technologies

2. Minimally Invasive and Targeted Therapies:

Surgery has traditionally been a treatment option for epilepsy, but minimally invasive techniques are emerging:

- Laser Ablation: This technique uses lasers to precisely target and destroy seizure-causing areas of the brain, offering a less invasive alternative to traditional surgery with faster recovery times.

- Refined Neuromodulation: Neuromodulation therapies like deep brain stimulation (DBS) and responsive neurostimulation (RNS) are being constantly improved. These devices can deliver targeted electrical stimulation to disrupt seizure activity.

- Closed-Loop Systems: Imagine a device implanted in your brain that can detect the beginning of a seizure and deliver a small electrical impulse to stop it before it even starts. Closed-loop systems are under development with the potential to be a game-changer for seizure control.

Part 5: The Future of Epilepsy Treatment
Chapter 12: Looking Ahead: Future Treatments and Technologies

3. Gene Therapy and the Power of Gene Editing:

The future of medicine might involve treating the root cause of diseases at the genetic level. This holds immense promise for epilepsy:

- Gene Therapy: This approach aims to deliver healthy genes to replace or repair faulty genes that contribute to epilepsy. While still in early stages, it has the potential to offer a long-term cure for some forms of the condition.

- Gene Editing: CRISPR-Cas9 gene editing technology is revolutionizing medicine. In theory, it could be used to modify genes associated with epilepsy, potentially offering a permanent solution in the future.

4. Improved Medications and Smarter Delivery Systems:

Medications are a mainstay of epilepsy treatment, and the future holds promise for even better options:

- New Anti-Seizure Medications: Research is ongoing to develop more effective medications with fewer side effects, allowing for better seizure control with a higher quality of life.

Part 5: The Future of Epilepsy Treatment
Chapter 12: Looking Ahead: Future Treatments and Technologies

- Targeted Drug Delivery: Scientists are exploring ways to deliver medications directly to the seizure focus in the brain. This targeted approach could minimize side effects on other parts of the body.

Looking Ahead:

It's important to remember that many of these advancements are still under investigation or in early development. However, the future of epilepsy treatment is undeniably bright. Here are some key takeaways:

- Individualized Treatment: The future of epilepsy treatment is moving towards personalized medicine, with treatment plans tailored to the specific type and cause of epilepsy in each individual.

- Continued Research is Crucial: Funding and research efforts are essential to bring these potential breakthroughs to fruition and improve the lives of people with epilepsy.

- Hope for a Brighter Future: The field of epilepsy treatment is constantly evolving, offering hope for a future where epilepsy can be effectively managed or even cured.

www.ingramcontent.com/pod-product-compliance
Lightning Source LLC
Chambersburg PA
CBHW071835210526
45479CB00001B/154